WONDERFUL BENEFITS OF FRUITS AND VEGETABLES

D. Stanly Kothem

TABLE OF CONTENTS

Chapter 1: REASONS WHY VITAMINS AND MINERALS ARE THE SOLUTION,

So many of us wish we had more energy, better abs, and more keen concentration. Similarly, we frequently wind up wishing that we would be advised to skin or hair. We wish that we could rest better around evening time, and wish that it was somewhat simpler to awaken (those last two focuses are connected, incidentally!).

This has prompted the development of various ventures, all worked around assisting us with feeling, look, and perform better. We burn through colossal measures of money on skincare items, on rest supplements, and on exercise center participations. We attempt a wide range of insane things, whether that is lying on a bed of delicate spikes to further develop rest (indeed, that is a genuine article!), wearing blue-impeding shades the entire day, or wearing energyhealing precious stones (which are comparably successful as wishing truly hard!).

We attempt these things since we're searching for replies, and we're frantic. We're willing to take a stab at anything. What's more, we trust, each time, that we're going to coincidentally find the response and open our maximum capacity.
We trust that ONE of these things will give the response and assist us with feeling Perfect as we realize that we truly can do. In any case, not many of these methodologies has any observable effect.

The issue? We're overcomplicating matters. What's more, this is generally because of the enormous measure of promoting that gets tossed at us consistently. In truth, further developing the manner in which you look and feel is extremely straightforward: it's about the rudiments!

Consider what is probably going to be your ongoing way of life and your ongoing eating routine. Lift your hand in the event that any of these focuses concern you:

* You don't deal with your five leafy foods daily
* You eat a great deal of handled food sources and prepared feasts
* You go to the exercise center 3 times each week or less - and aren't especially portable the remainder of the time
* You don't get sufficient rest
* You are in a condition of constant pressure because of work, family, and monetary tensions
* You spend a great deal of your spare energy on the sofa, watching kid's shows
* You spend over eight hours daily taking a gander at a PC screen, with a slouched back, gazing at a splendid screen
* You invest scarcely any energy outside
* You drink polluted regular water
* You inhale destructive exhaust cloud filled air

This is a somewhat disheartening picture, however it's valid for The overwhelming majority of us. We don't eat an adequate number of greens, we don't rest, we gorge on sweet food varieties, and we're focused on constantly. Then we can't help thinking about why we don't feel 100 percent!

Regardless of whether you got the vast majority of these things right, truly our advanced ways of life are only totally horrendous for our wellbeing.

This is valid directly down to the way that a large portion of us are excessively agreeable - we have become "adjusted" to an agreeable, trained way of life, and consequently our bodies have failed to remember how to manage pressure or trouble.

Take going outside for example. The vast majority of us simply don't do sufficiently this, and that implies that we aren't getting the significant boost of daylight, which assists with empowering the body to create vitamin D, which thus controls things like chemical creation, rest, temperament... even craving!

Without that significant info (called an "outside zeitgebers" in the logical writing) our body loses a portion of its normal beat and certain cycles are interfered.

However at that point there's the gigantic advantage of being vulnerable. In any event, when the sun isn't out, being outside assists with helping testosterone levels, fortify our resistant framework, and even work on our capacity to direct our own internal heat level.

Is anyone surprised we generally feel "stodgy" when we never train this piece of our wellbeing?

In any event, investing energy barefooted on the earth (which trains small muscles in the foot), in any event, plunging into water and pausing our breathing (which prepares our lungs and further develops our CO2 balance)... these are everything our bodies desire. Also, we aren't giving them that.

What's more, our bodies are decaying greatly therefore. Contrast a wolf in the wild with an overweight, ruined homegrown canine. Which is better?

YOU are that homegrown canine. In addition a very upsetting way of life and absence of rest...

THE SOLUTION IS To START WITH FRUITS AND VEGETABLES

Beginning with vegetables and organic products is the arrangement. Why?

All things considered, it's all awesome and well me letting you know that you ought to be resolving over the course of the day, and that you ought to eat impeccably, and that you ought to be taking long swims in freezing cold water in the first part of the day. Issue is, we lack the capacity to deal with that and our bodies are currently maladapted to such an extent that they wouldn't deal with it.

In any event, fixing your eating regimen - disposing of all that undesirable handled food, decreasing the quantity of complete calories, getting more fiber, lessening basic carbs… it's a lo of work and can get very muddled. Which is the reason the best spot to begin is by fixing one of the greatest issues with current life. That is: the absence of micronutrients.

Micronutrients are nutrients, minerals, amino acids, unsaturated fats, cell reinforcements, and other dynamic fixings in our food that our body utilizes for a wide range of purposes.

What many individuals don't understand is that we in a real sense are what we eat. You hear this a ton, yet many individuals expect that it is a sort of representation. Yet, no: your body takes in the supplements that you consume and afterward it utilizes those supplements to modify your body as a matter of fact.

For instance, your bones are made part of the way from calcium, and magnesium. These likewise help to reinforce your connective tissue (ligaments and tendons), your teeth, and your nails. Connective tissues likewise benefit from any semblance of collagen (tracked down in bone stock) which additionally assists with working on your skin.

If by some stroke of good luck you could get more leafy foods in your eating regimen then, at that point, you would turn into the best and best variant of yourself. Furthermore, that thus could then give you the energy and self discipline to wrap up.

Foods grown from the ground might supercharge your digestion, assisting you with consuming substantially more fat!

As we will find in the remainder of this book, fixing your admission of foods grown from the ground needn't bother with to be troublesome. In the event that you are vital, simplifying only a couple of changes can change your wellbeing and prosperity.

This book will likewise frame a significant number of the other astounding and complex manners by which organic products can work on your wellbeing and execution - some of which are totally extraordinary to the manner in which you look and feel.

You'll know exactly which products of the soil you really want to fix any of your ongoing diseases, and you'll know definitively how to get them.

CHAPTER 2: **INTRODUCTION TO VITAMINS**

Before we go further, we should analyze all the more intently the particular advantages of foods grown from the ground. Furthermore, obviously, the primary spot to begin is by taking a gander at the nutrient substance.

It might amaze you to realize that nutrients were found under a long time back. Until they were authoritatively found, specialists realize that specific food sources assisted with specific states of being, however they didn't have the foggiest idea why.

For instance, the English Naval force conveyed a stockpile of limes as soon as 1975 on the grounds that specialists had tracked down that eating a specific sum every day, or drinking the juice, prevented mariners from getting scurvy.

Nonetheless, it was only after 1912 that Casimir Funk, working in the UK afterward in the USA thought of the expression "vitamines," which later became nutrients.
The investigation of nutrients has advanced since that time, and though the vast majority of us know the names of the most widely recognized nutrients, we may not necessarily comprehend what they do. There are two sorts of nutrients. These are fat dissolvable nutrients and water solvent nutrients.

Fat dissolvable nutrients are those nutrients that the body can store. This intends that on the off chance that you don't utilize every one of the nutrients that you consume, they can be put away in the body for use when the body is needing them.

The conspicuous benefit of fat solvent nutrients is that in the event that your eating regimen is briefly ailing in one of these nutrients, you are less inclined to experience a lack. That weakness of these sorts of nutrients is that on the off chance that you consume a lot of one of them, your body can't flush out the excess and you could experience the ill effects of a nutrient excess.

Fat Dissolvable Nutrients

The most regularly realized fat solvent nutrients are vitamin A, vitamin D, vitamin E and vitamin K.

Vitamin An assists with keeping the skin saturated, as well as guaranteeing that the bodily fluid films stay clammy, flexible and smooth. It additionally assists with keeping up with solid vision in low light, as well as keeping the regenerative framework sound and advancing solid bone development. Wellsprings of vitamin An incorporate entire milk, margarine, eggs and liver. A type of vitamin A, carotenoids are tracked down in red, yellow and dim green vegetables and organic product.

Vitamin D is fundamental for the body to assimilate calcium. Hence, it is answerable for solid teeth and bones, very much like calcium. Notwithstanding, both are required and cooperate. Vitamin D is frequently added to 'braced' food sources like fat spreads and grains. It is otherwise called the daylight nutrient as the principal wellspring of vitamin D comes from daylight.

Vitamin E is answerable for keeping up with solid muscles, sensory system and conceptive framework. It is additionally an enemy of oxidant. Being fat dissolvable, it is put away in the body and can assist with safeguarding body cells from the impacts of free extremists, which be harming to other body cells.

Wellsprings of vitamin E incorporate entire grains, nuts, raw grain oil and green verdant vegetables. Ingesting too much nutrient is believed to be hazardous. Vitamin K is predominantly liable for blood thickening. Without it, each time you cut yourself you would be at risk for draining to death.

This nutrient additionally makes kidney tissues and bone. Wellsprings of vitamin K incorporate liver, cheddar, oats, dim green verdant vegetables and natural product. It is additionally made in the digestion tracts by amicable microscopic organisms.

Water solvent nutrients can't be put away in the body. This actually intends that assuming you consume a lot of one of these nutrients, the sum that isn't utilized is discharged through pee. The benefit of water solvent nutrients is that you are probably not going to experience the ill effects of an excess.

The detriment of these nutrients is that you might have to accept in bigger sums as it can't be put away. On the off chance that your eating regimen is lacking in one of these nutrients, in any event, for a brief time frame, you might endure side effects of lack of nutrient thus, there is no back up supply put away in your body.

Water Solvent Nutrients

The most ordinarily realize water solvent nutrients are L-ascorbic acid, and the whole gathering of B nutrients. L-ascorbic acid is otherwise called ascorbic corrosive. It assists with keeping up with the body's connective tissues, or at least, the muscle, fat, and bone structure.

It additionally assists with mending wounds by accelerating the development of new cells, is an enemy of oxidant, and assists the body with engrossing iron. One more capability of L-ascorbic acid is to safeguard the body's resistant framework empowering it to battle contamination.

Wellsprings of L-ascorbic acid incorporate natural product, organic product juices and vegetables. The B gathering of nutrients comprises of B1 or thiamin, B2 or riboflavin, B3 or niacin, B6 or pyridoxine and B12 or cyanocobalamin. This gathering of nutrients is basically worried about keeping the body working appropriately.

Vitamin B1 is fundamental in assisting the body with processing energy from fats, liquor and carbs. Wellsprings of this nutrient are lean pork, crude cereals, seeds and nuts.

B2 assists the body with utilizing and digest starches and proteins and keeps a sound hunger. Wellsprings of B2 incorporate fish, poultry, meat, milk and eggs. Brewers yeast is a decent wellspring of this nutrient, as are dull verdant vegetables.

B3 is fundamental for appropriate development and empowering oxygen to move through body tissues. It is likewise liable for keeping a solid craving. Wellsprings of vitamin B3 incorporate braced bread and oats and meat.

B6 is answerable for acquiring supplements and energy from the food we eat. It forestalls coronary illness by eliminating overabundance homocysteine from the blood. Wellsprings of B6 incorporate soya beans, implies, nuts, eggs, entire grains, fish, sheep, port, chicken and milk.

B12 assists with making solid red platelets. It additionally empowers the body to communicate messages between the body's nerve cells, empowering us to hear, move, think and ordinary regular exercises. It is made by microbes in the body's small digestive system.

This nutrient is added to numerous food varieties, including oats, and despite the fact that it is a water solvent nutrient, it tends to be put away in the liver. Wellsprings of B12 includepoultry, fish, milk, meat and eggs.

The most effective way of guaranteeing that you take in an adequate number of water solvent and fat dissolvable nutrients is to eat a reasonable eating regimen. On the off chance that you feel that you might be lacking in certain nutrients, you ought to counsel a specialist for guidance.

CHAPTER 3: **INSTRUCTION TO MINERALS AND OTHER ASTONISHING SUPPLEMENTS IN PRODUCTS OF THE SOIL**

While organic products are regularly loaded with nutrients, minerals will generally come moreso from our vegetables - however no doubt about it, the two leafy foods are loaded with both.

All in all, a decent inquiry to begin with may be: what is the distinction between a nutrient and a mineral?

While nutrients are natural and in this manner are ordinarily very unstable (they can be separated by any semblance of intensity, air, and corrosive), minerals are on the other hand inorganic. Truth be told, a mineral can truly be a metal or a stone - something you could never truly consider being a crucial structure block in what makes you.
In any case, to be sure minerals are essential to the solid capability of the human body. Iron for instance is an essential mineral that the body uses to make hemoglobin - the red platelets that movement around the body conveying oxygen.

Without this cycle, it would be difficult to give energy around the body to the innumerable urgent capabilities that go on - including breathing, processing, from there, the sky is the limit.

Regularly, minerals will generally have a somewhat more central job in the underlying components of the human body - and the harder components. For instance, minerals structure bones, ligaments, and tendons.

Minerals likewise assume a part in conduction, be that as it may. The body is fueled by power all things considered, and keeping up with the right charge is essential for the solid capability of our muscles and mind.

That is the reason an inaccurate equilibrium between sodium and potassium can cause squeezing, as the body can't send messages accurately to the muscles. In like manner, an absence of calcium can diminish strength as dealing with the charge in the muscle cells is required.

Did you be aware? You can differentiate between a foods grown from the ground in view of the seed/stone. Vegetables don't have them! Food sources that have astounding orders include: tomatoes (organic product), coconut (organic product), avocado (organic product), and cucumber (organic product).
Other Fundamental Micronutrients

As well as being plentiful in nutrients and minerals, foods grown from the ground are likewise a rich wellspring of the two other fundamental supplements. The other fundamental supplements are: fundamental unsaturated fats, and fundamental amino acids.

The expression "fundamental" implies that these substances can't be blended inside the body, thus in this way should be gotten from our eating routine. What's more, maybe this ought to likewise be a sign concerning how large an issue it is that the vast majority of us are not getting them that way!

Anyway, what do these supplements do?

Indeed, amino acids are basically the structure blocks of proteins. We get a ton of these from meat, and our bodies will then separate those constituent parts to reconstruct our tissue. As we saw toward the beginning of this book, we in a real sense are what we eat!

For this reason amino acids and proteins likewise are so significant for weight lifters and competitors attempting to fabricate muscle.

Research proposes that the ideal equilibrium for competitors is 1 gram of protein for each 1lb of bodyweight. Protein likewise has different advantages - it is a lot harder to change over into fat for example, and it has a thermogenic impact implying that essentially processing it will really consume calories!

In this manner, many individuals will be working diligently attempting to find wellsprings of protein from meat and will eat a lot of chicken to fabricate greater muscles. This can turn out to be difficult work! Yet, what they neglect is that vegetables and even organic products additionally contain protein (however vegetables are marginally predominant in this sense).

Try not to simply count the protein you got from that protein shake and chicken, contemplate how much is in the broccoli on the chicken.

Amino acids likewise play a large group of different jobs in the body and are utilized to create stomach related compounds, synapses (mind synthetic substances) and considerably more. They can likewise do things, for example, making.

At long last, products of the soil contain fundamental unsaturated fats. These are significant fats that assist us with bettering retain different foods grown from the ground, and furthermore serve a scope of extra helpful advantages -, for example, improving mind capability (the cerebrum is made of a lot of fat!).

Omega 3 is quite possibly of the most remarkable fundamental unsaturated fat there is and has a Gigantic host of astonishing advantages. Frequently, we consider omega 3 being something we get from fish, however truth be told it additionally exists in great sums in ocean growth, hemp seed, pecans, kidney beans, soybean and that's only the tip of the iceberg.

Chapter 4: LEAFY FOODS FOR ATHLETIC EXECUTION

At the point when you consider an eating regimen for building muscle, your brain presumably goes to the exemplary choices. You probably will zero in basically on protein sources like chicken, fish and eggs. A competitor's eating regimen ought to comprise of only meta and steamed rice, correct?

Yet, this is a long way from the main sort of food that will be helpful for building muscle and further developing execution. Truth be told, for working out, running, swimming, significant distance running, and some other sort of athletic pursuit you really should get a fair eating routine that will consolidate an extensive variety of various nutritional categories. Specifically, it is significant you get your leafy foods. Keen on taking enhancements to help your athletic exhibition? What could intrigue you to learn is that consuming leafy foods can really be more compelling while likewise costing significantly less and having a bunch of other astonishing medical advantages!

Here are a few models.

Top Foods grown from the ground That Work on Athletic Execution

Beets

Beets are by a long shot among the exceptionally most significant vegetables for building muscle and for competitors, everything being equal.

That is on the grounds that beets are among the best food sources on the planet with regards to raising nitric oxide. Nitric oxide is a characteristic 'vasodilator'. This implies that it can cause the veins (veins and supply routes) to expand (extend) subsequently reassuring the progression of oxygen and supplements around the body.

The outcome is that the muscles get more oxygen and energy during preparing and more supplements for upgrading recuperation. This can assist you with lifting for additional reps, run further distances and recuperate at a quicker rate.

Potatoes

Sugars are frequently portrayed as the miscreants yet truth be told they are vital for building muscle and for actual preparation overall. Potatoes are a decent decision of sugar since they're likewise high in fiber, high in L-ascorbic acid (which improves recuperation) and low in calories. Consume after an exercise and the energy will go directly to the muscles instead of the midsection.
Spinach

Spinach is a vegetable that is high in protein as well similar to a decent wellspring of phytoecdysteroids. These share nothing practically speaking with anabolic steroids except for they might make a comparative difference
- for certain examinations recommending they are a decent choice for empowering muscle building and testosterone creation.

Kale

Kale is the vegetable most elevated in calcium. Calcium is very significant for your exercises, in addition to the fact that it assists with reinforcing the bones however it likewise builds up your connective tissue and it assists with fortifying compressions for more dangerous power during exercises.

Kale is extremely stylish right currently being high in protein and low in calories. However, a disgrace it costs a fair piece!

Mushrooms

Mushrooms are in fact not natural products or vegetables, but rather they are found in a similar passageway and they're ok for vegetarians, so they're fair game to incorporate here. Mushrooms are one more extraordinary wellspring of protein as well as accompanied an extensive variety of extra medical advantages and benefits. They're loaded with minerals, they can energize recuperation from preparing and substantially more close to!

It's inevitable until we begin seeing mushroom protein shakes springing up in wellbeing stores!

The other astonishing advantage of mushrooms is that they contain vitamin D. Truth be told, they're one of a handful of the dietary wellsprings of vitamin D! (Another being slick fish).
This is significant seeing as vitamin D is viewed as an expert chemical controller, and is liable for empowering the creation of testosterone specifically - one of the vitally anabolic chemicals for building muscle and consuming fat.

Furthermore, is that vitamin D has as of late been demonstrated to be significantly more powerful than even L-ascorbic acid with regards to supporting the safe framework and forestalling colds and sicknesses. As any competitor knows, a virus can be sufficient to finish wreck and competitors preparing plan, which thus can be the contrast among triumph and disappointment!

Carrots

Carrots are for the most part solid and an incredible wellspring of vitamin A, C and K. What's truly interesting about them however is the lutein, which might assist with expanding energy levels and upgrade the proficiency of your very mitochondria!

Your mitochondria are the energy plants of your cells which convert glucose into ATP (glucose being the sugar that comes from carbs, and ATP being the usable type of energy in your body). This in short intends that with carrots and different wellsprings of lutein, you can really run quicker and that you'll truly consume more calories in any event, while you're resting!

In one review, rodents were given lutein (which needs a wellspring of fat to retain like milk) and it was found that they started running significant distances willfully in their wheel, consuming considerably more fat as they did.

Apples

Apples are plentiful in L-ascorbic acid, which is one more essential nutrient for improving the resistant framework and assisting competitors with preparing longer and harder as a matter of course. L-ascorbic acid additionally assists with empowering the maintenance of muscle tissue, expands serotonin to help with mental recuperation, and even builds the development of both testosterone and nitric oxide when matched with zinc.

On top of this, apples are likewise exceptionally wealthy in fiber, which can assist with further developing defecations, the retention of food, pulse, and that's just the beginning. Fiber is likewise key to supporting a sound microbiome, which thus can uphold a solid invulnerable framework, better mind-set, weight reduction, and substantially more.

Chapter 5: **ASTOUNDING SUPERFOOD PRODUCTS OF THE SOIL FOR STATE of MIND, ENERGY, MAGNIFICENCE, AND THAT'S JUST THE BEGINNING**

Anyway, you're not especially keen on weight reduction? Maybe you are now content with the size you are? (Congrats!)

Perhaps you're not a competitor? Perhaps you don't have recognizable medical conditions?

See, foods grown from the ground are for everybody. Furthermore, just to slam that point home, here are a few additional instances of foods grown from the ground with ridiculously fluctuating different sound advantages
Broccoli and Mixed Greens for Excellence and Pregnancy

Indeed, products of the soil can assist with making you look more gorgeous. What's more, that is valid even of something as basic as your unassuming broccoli!

Broccoli is maybe somewhat less 'extraordinary' when contrasted and a portion of the other superfood products of the soil on this rundown. In any case, don't let that fool you: this is as yet an unbelievably nutritious food that everybody ought to get a greater amount of.

Yet again first off, broccoli is a decent wellspring of fiber and can assist with working on your processing, your solid discharges, and considerably more. In addition however, broccoli is likewise extremely high in nutrients K, L-ascorbic acid, fiber, potassium, collagen, iron, calcium, and that's just the beginning.

How about we start by plunging into that collagen. This is the kind of thing that we all need however not very many of us get. Collagen has been displayed to further develop cerebrum capability and battle against Alzheimer's, it additionally assists with decreasing back torment, further develops skin flexibility, fortifies the nails, battles flawed stomach condition, battles knee torment, and for the most part strengthens your ligaments, tendons, and bones.

To this end feasts, for example, bone stock as so amazingly really great for us. Furthermore, presently late examination is proposing a much more impressive explanation that collagen may be so significant. Analysts presently suspect that people would whenever have lived basically by eating bone marrow from creature cadavers. The contention goes that huntergatherers might have been unprepared to take on huge prey. Be that as it may, we were truly adept at finding our prey and following them.

What probably would have happened frequently, is that we would have followed impalas and different creatures to the place where they were gone after and killed by creatures like lions and tigers. They would then have stripped those creatures of all their meat, abandoning the skeleton. That is the point at which the cleverness and creative people would have gone along, torn open the bones with our material hands, and afterward eaten the nutritious collagen from inside.
On the off chance that this is for sure obvious, we advanced in a climate where we consumed a lot of the constituents of bone. Furthermore, we presently wind up flung into a reality where we seldom get these significant supplements. In the event that that is the situation, broccoli might be much more gainful than we at first expected!

Pregnant moms ought to investigate eating more broccoli and more greens overall. That is on the grounds that both broccoli and numerous plate of mixed greens leaves are a decent wellspring of folate, which is something that all moms are prescribed to eat.

Not getting sufficient folate expands the gamble of difficulties in pregnancy, and that is the reason a great deal of moms will attempt to get all the more misleadingly using pregnancy supplements.

This is where it means quite a bit to bring up the huge benefits of getting a greater number of supplements from your eating routine as opposed to from supplements. While it is actually the case that you can profit from supplements, the educate here is the name. These are planned to enhance your standard eating regimen.

In other words that they ought to be taken notwithstanding your ordinary eating routine, as opposed to as another option. Supplements from your eating routine are definitely more powerful than those taken in pill structure, as they are joined with various different supplements, fats, filaments, and different components.

Together, these assistance to further develop ingestion of the critical components and that makes them considerably more successful. What to perceive is that the human body developed while being presented to these food varieties and subsequently is ideally intended to separate the dietary benefit here.

Consuming supplements in a manufactured form isn't planned. This is the reason so many tell you not to take nutrient tablets while starving'. They simply work better as food varieties.

Cayenne Pepper for Weight reduction, Testosterone, and the sky is the limit from there

Cayenne pepper in the mean time is one more extraordinary device in the fight against irritation. This is a compound that makes food fiery and is broadly tracked down in treatments and creams because of its enemy of irritation impacts. It's a typical painrelief too as it exhausts nerve cells of the compound 'substance P'. Substance P causes both irritation and the impression of torment, so this is something incredible to add to your eating routine on the off chance that you truly do experience the ill effects of a condition like fibromyalgia or joint inflammation.

Cayenne additionally comes loaded with flavonoids and carotenoids. These are cancer prevention agents that forestall cell harm, in this way further battling against irritation.

Cayenne pepper likewise has various other noteworthy advantages. It has been demonstrated to be a compelling craving suppressant for example, intending that assuming you are somebody who battles to adhere to an eating routine, you could begin viewing it somewhat simpler as focused and in this way ideally see the weight start to tumble off.

Simultaneously, cayenne pepper might assist with further developing processing. This is significant in light of the fact that better assimilation doesn't just give you more energy and forestall distress, yet it likewise assists you with bettering retain supplements from your food. That implies that every one of the advantages you're getting from the other superfoods on this rundown will then, at that point, be gone up to 11.

What's more is that cayenne pepper has likewise been displayed to increment testosterone. This obviously is the chemical that the greater part of us know as the 'male chemical' and is answerable for the male sex

drive, as well as a large number of the distinctions among people. Expanding testosterone in men increments muscle tone, diminishes fat capacity, raises animosity, helps with recuperation, sustains the resistant framework and that's only the tip of the iceberg.
Men who don't get sufficient testosterone will display indications of misery, low energy, low state of mind, and low sex drive. They likewise battle with weight gain and low bulk. Alternately, men with high testosterone show the attributes that we partner with the exemplary 'dominant man' alongside conditioned and strong constitutions.

This is the reason such countless men attempt to increase their normal testosterone creation using steroids and different medications - notwithstanding those conveying various wellbeing admonitions and serious risks.

The truly stressing part is that testosterone in men is expanding across the globe by 1% per year. This is halfway because of the utilization of female items and their effect on our water, alongside a large group of different issues (certain plastics and our for the most part inert ways of life). Yet, diet has a Major impact in it as well. Time to begin eating somewhat less handled food, and somewhat more cayenne pepper.

Elderberry for Irritation

Elderberry is a berry that is wealthy in supplements. Once more a natural product is missing from a large number of our ordinary weight control plans, as it's one that you ought to consider once again introducing.

The straightforward truth is that the greater part of us depend on similar few products of the soil every day of the week. Along these lines however, we are guaranteeing we get a ton of supplements as a result, while passing up some others. The best eating regimen is the most changed diet - the one that incorporates the greatest scope of various natural products, vegetables, meats, spices, and the sky is the limit from there. So how might elderberry at any point help you?

Elderberry has been utilized since ancient times and has been utilized as an enhancement or medication by a large group of old societies - including the Old Egyptians. Today we currently realize that these organic products are amazingly high in flavonoids and particularly our companions anthocyanins - strong cell reinforcements like resveratrol.
Simultaneously, elderberries have been displayed to assist with helping the development of cytokines. These are the courier particles that our bodies use to control the invulnerable framework. Ace fiery cytokines help to support irritation, while mitigating cytokines help to decrease them. This is all vital in light of the fact that it essentially guarantees that the body can appropriately direct its own reaction to infections and sicknesses, and to assist with mending wounds and wounds.

Large numbers of us imagine that irritation is generally something terrible - as a matter of fact however, irritation assists with obliterating contaminations before they get an opportunity to produce results, as well as to support recuperating by conveying more supplements to the impacted region. The issue is the point at which this reaction goes haywire.

It would seem for comparative reasons, elderberry could likewise be profoundly viable at fighting sensitivities!

On top of this, elderberries are likewise exceptionally compelling at battling and obliterating microorganisms, being valuable in battling contaminations, colds, and a large group of different issues.

Generally intriguing of all, the small berries contain intense antiviral specialists that have been displayed to really 'deactivate' infections.

These work by forestalling the infections from having the option to get through cell walls utilizing their haemagglutinin spikes, which thusly delivers them practically dormant. They are accordingly exceptionally powerful for battling issues like rhinitis, as well as keeping them from happening in any case.

Obviously, there is additionally the typical nutrient and mineral substance that you will generally get from it

Chapter 6: HOW CELL REINFORCEMENTS ASSIST YOU WITH LIVING LONGER

Cell reinforcements are tracked down normally in our eating routine and are likewise a critical component of numerous enhancements. Cell reinforcements are something of a trendy expression nowadays and cancer prevention agent nutrients and minerals as well as a scope of Naka Spice supplements are profoundly famous.

What is the justification for this? Furthermore, what unequivocally are cancer prevention agents? Here we will look a little at how a cell functions, how a cell kicks the bucket and why cell reinforcements are so significant.

Our cells are comprised of different parts yet all you want to realize about this occasion is the cell wall and the core. The cell wall, encompassed by mitochondria, is the piece of the cell that obviously keeps it all intact and gives the cell its round appearance.
In the meantime the core is the focal point of the cell, which is frequently alluded to as the 'control focus'. In here is where the DNA is put away, the 'plan' that lets the cell know what it resembles, how to act and where the other significant cells go in the body.

Tragically however what's likewise in our body is 'free revolutionaries' and this is where the cell reinforcement nutrients and minerals and the Naka Spice supplements come in. Basically free extremists are substances that move around the body and harm the phones. They are a side-effect of numerous things from essentially breathing (oxygen is receptive and harms cells) to getting an excess of direct daylight (the UV waves in the daylight are radioactive and can harm our cell walls as well).

These free revolutionaries then cause a ton of serious harm in the body and are sufficient to ultimately make our skin look more seasoned - in light of the fact that the harm however minute can ultimately amount to be noticeable to the unaided eye and this goes for skin cells too. To this end heaps of openness to the sun will do right by you and tanned for the time being, in any case bring about your skin seeming crumpled and weathered.

All the more genuinely however, at last these free extremists will break the whole way through the cell walls, and this will imply that they arrive at the core where the DNA is housed. In the event that they arrive at this, they can make harm your really hereditary code and this results in a transformation which changes the declaration of the cell and renders it unfit to take care of its business.

Since cells replicate by parting (mitosis) this then implies that when the cell parts it will duplicate the DNA across and you will have two issue cells. Your invulnerable framework attempts to stop this and can be helped in the event that you purchase spices on the web, however it would be better obviously on the off chance that it very well may be forestalled. Since those dead cells as they spread become disease, and can ultimately prompt the disappointment of entire organs.

Cell reinforcement nutrients and minerals from organic products, vegetables, and even enhancements will assist you with doing this - by annihilating the free revolutionaries on influence accordingly forestalling them truly causing that harm. These will then sluggish your apparent maturing and assist with preventing malignant growth - not terrible!

Chapter 7: **HOW TO UTILIZE PRODUCTS OF THE SOIL TO FURTHER DEVELOP YOUR WELL BEING EFFECTIVELY**

Right now, you ought to have an extensive thought of the best motivations to guarantee you are getting an adequate number of products of the soil in your eating routine. These can improve your wellbeing in a heap ways, and in the event that you are right now feeling drained, cranky, unwell, or even discouraged, almost certainly, you have a lack in something like one of these micronutrients. Also, this ought to shock no one - considering that by far most of individuals In all actuality do have a lack these days of some sort.

The following inquiry is the way you ought to be tenderly coordinating these foods grown from the ground. Are there any downsides? What number of do you want unequivocally? Might you at any point utilize a nutrient tablet all things being equal?

What number of Products of the soil Do You Really want Truly?

You could have heard that you ought to expect to consume something like five distinct products of the soil a day. This is a piece of general counsel that is given by numerous wellbeing associations and legislatures. A few associations have expanded this number to seven. It is solid counsel, but it is additionally inconsistent.

What do I mean by that? Basically, that it depends on nothing!

Leafy foods are not intrinsically great for you. They are not really great for you since they are leafy foods. Rather, they are really great for you Since they contain that large number of fundamental micronutrients.

Those micronutrients are expected in various amounts and assortments, and at last the smartest option for our wellbeing is simply to get however many of them as could be allowed. The more products of the soil you consume, the better. Also, it is extremely difficult to go too far when you get your supplements from regular sources like this.

Furthermore, be extremely questionable when a bundle of food lets you know it considers "one of your five every day." On the off chance that that food is profoundly handled, odds are it will not contain numerous supplements in it by any means any longer. In any event, being a lot of lower in fiber is probable.

In this way, the advantages will not be all around as extraordinary as they would have been had you consumed that supplement itself. Apply some sound judgment, and where conceivable, eat as some entire, genuine foods grown from the ground as you can!

The Risks of Such a large number of Products of the soil

All things considered, you can cause yourself harm by consuming such a large number of products of the soil. Or on the other hand to be somewhat more unambiguous, it is generally simple to hurt by consuming a lot of natural product.

That is on the grounds that organic product is exceptionally acidic and loaded with sugar. Both these things make it harming to your teeth specifically. Many individuals who change to slims down that are fundamentally focussed on the utilization of smoothies will wind up creating serious tooth issues!

One answer for this is to try not to drink a lot of natural product juice or too many natural product smoothies. All things considered, center around drinking vegetable smoothies, which ordinarily contain much less sugar.

Another thought is that leafy foods are as yet a wellspring of calories. This is particularly valid for things like avocados, which have turned into extremely popular as of late. While avocados are perfect for supporting testosterone (on account of their solid soaked fat substance), and keeping in mind that they are helpful for those attempting to stay away from carbs, they can in any case make you fat!

Try not to wrongly imagine that "leafy foods are sound and in this manner can't make you fat."

Truly they actually contain calories you actually need to follow and deal with those calories to stay away from undesirable weight gain.

Chapter 8: **MAKING AN EATING REGIMEN WEALTHY IN LEAFY FOODS**

In this way, you should eat more products of the soil, and we've seen currently that there are countless explicit food sources that have an especially great advantage - similarly as there are an immense number of explicit nutrients and minerals that you want to attempt to search out in your eating regimen.

In any case, how would you approach executing that arrangement? How would you go from attempting to get your five per day, to having the option to consume an enormous plenty of various valuable fixings without any problem?

Since that is the other key thing to understand: you ought not be adopting a reductive strategy of attempting to independently search out every thing. On the off chance that you do this, you'll find that you wind up burning through an enormous measure of cash, and at last not getting a lot of advantage. This book has recorded an enormous number of products of the soil that you can search out explicitly to appreciate benefits for your excellence, for your energy levels, for irritation, for invulnerability... You could subsequently be enticed to figure you can single out the advantages you need! However, this is some unacceptable methodology.

At the point when there are THAT a wide range of superfoods that each proposition some sort of astounding advantage, you can't search out every one independently. This is particularly evident considering large numbers of them won't combine as one, many aren't accessible in your neighborhood general store, and some may be consumable for a short measure of time. Anyway, what do you do all things considered?

The Methodology: The Point is Assortment

Rather than searching out individual various foods grown from the ground, what is far ideal is to just plan to get the greatest assortment you can in your eating regimen. By doing this, you will cover the biggest range of fixings, and subsequently get the biggest scope of various advantages from your eating routine.

You could find the best superfood vegetable on the planet, yet in the event that that was all you ate then you wouldn't get all that much advantage - in light of the fact that you'd just be getting a lot of those equivalent fixings.

We don't consider food sources, for example, apples as being super food sources, but since they contain a lot of L-ascorbic acid (cell reinforcement, helps testosterone, supports nitric oxide development, produces serotonin), epicatechin, they are similarly essentially as great as those more colorful thoughts.

In addition, on the off chance that you eat three unique foods grown from the ground, the scope of supplements you get will be far more noteworthy.

Concentrates on show too, that our microbiome - the solid microorganisms living in our guts - benefit in particular from a changed eating routine. The more noteworthy the scope of food sources you eat, the more grounded your stomach wellbeing will be - bringing about weight reduction, more energy, better state of mind, and that's only the tip of the iceberg.

At last, by expecting to simply "eat loads of products of the soil" you can diminish how much thought this diet support includes, which thus will assist you with being bound to adhere to your new responsibility.

Step by step instructions to Expand The Range of Organic products and Vegetables

So how would you build the assortment? Here are a few simple tips that will assist you with doing that without adding a ton of stress to your next shopping trip:

• Make loads of stews, hot pots, and Italian dishes. In the event that you're cooking something like a bolognaise, it's quite simple to toss a lot of products of the soil into a pot with some mince.

• To make this significantly simpler, have a go at grinding things like carrot (so you don't have to strip), and utilize frozen fixings like mushrooms, peas, and sweetcorn.

• Make bunches of plates of mixed greens! A simple method for making a virus lunch is to get some plate of mixed greens leaves, toss on a few yams, cut some cucumber, and add a spot of lemon. This can go on almost ANYTHING you cook. Pick child leaf spinach and you'll get iron and folate. Then fluctuate which leaf you utilize without fail.

• Hold up! While doing this, concoct enormous groups of food varieties and afterward freeze them in loads of exclusively partitioned tupperwares. Then all you really want to do is to thaw out every one as you come to eat it.

• Make smoothies! These are very simple to create - toss a lot of leafy foods/vegetables in and hit mix. They likewise give an immense increase in astonishing advantages. Probably the most vigorous and blissful individuals I know consume everyday smoothies!

• Purchase foods grown from the ground out. A great deal of bistros sell natural products at the counter, and the equivalent is valid in numerous merchants. Rather than purchasing a chocolatey nibble, simply purchase the most colorful looking natural product you can find!

Chapter 9: **WHAT MIGHT BE SAID ABOUT MULTIVITAMIN ENHANCEMENTS?**

In the event that the fundamental advantages of products of the soil come from the nutrients, minerals, and other fundamental micronutrients, then you could have an entirely sensible inquiry: what might be said about multivitamins?

A multivitamin supplement is an enhancement that contains an equilibrium of various supplements. You could normally see one that contains a mix of L-ascorbic acid, D, A, and B complex. Moreover, multimineral enhancements could contain Iron, Magnesium, Potassium, Calcium, and Zinc for "solid bones and chemical equilibrium."

Are these items comparably great as the "genuine article?"

Indeed and negative.
From one viewpoint, you can assimilate and profit from supplements. Certain individuals will let you know that this isn't correct, yet there are a few valid justifications to accept in any case. As far as one might be concerned, did you had at least some idea that there really exist a few items that are intended to supplant your whole eating routine? These incorporate any semblance of Soylent, which apparently contains each and every supplement the body needs, all fair impeccably.

Is it a smart thought? Not the slightest bit! In any case, what to zero in on right presently is that individuals who utilize this item get by… and they're quite solid! Furthermore, in view of that, we can thusly state without a doubt that multivitamins can likewise be consumed.

Be that as it may, there's a trick. The first of these gets is that a multivitamin is simply going to be pretty much as great as the individual who planned it. We saw with lutein and other fatsoluble nutrients for instance. These need a wellspring of fat to be retained into the circulation system. Get them from regular food sources, and odds are good that the wellspring of fat will be incorporated. Get them from a nutrient enhancement and they could not.

Comparable collaborations likewise exist between numerous different nutrients and minerals, where one will help the other to effectively be ingested more. Moreover, various nutrients and minerals ingest at various rates, thus preferably ought not be joined into a solitary item.

Then, at that point, there are different things that leafy foods contain that do us great - like fiber, amino acids, and that's just the beginning. Also there's the little reality that all foods grown from the ground contain substances that we don't completely have any idea or maybe aren't even mindful of.

We just barely found the uncommon advantages of lutein (that go past eye wellbeing). So eating genuine leafy foods is Consistently best.

In any case, so, in the event that the decision comes down to utilizing an enhancement or not getting those valuable supplements by any stretch of the imagination… then, at that point, the enhancement is obviously better. As a matter of fact, an enhancement can be an exceptionally helpful and simple method for getting what you want in your eating routine, or can be viewed as a "back up."

Chapter 10: **CONCLUSION - YOUR DIAGRAM FOR MORE PROMINENT WELL-BEING**

What's more, with that, we arrive at the finish of this aide. As of now, you ought to now have a vastly improved thought of unequivocally which leafy foods you want in your eating routine, which ones can give the most advantages, and how really the range of these things bests all the other things.

Similarly, you ought to now have a comprehension of the most ideal ways to get those leafy foods in your eating routine, and the most effective ways to stay away from any issues that can emerge out of them.

With everything that expressed, here is your outline to help your wellbeing and joy greatly by getting more products of the soil:

- Begin your day with a smoothie, yet don't have more than one organic product smoothie

- Try not to mean to get only 5-7 products of the soil in your eating regimen. Set the most that you can up to get a shifted blend.

- Utilize an enhancement as a "back up." This is likewise particularly helpful while searching out additional dark and interesting supplements.

- In any case, ensure that you read the directions and do your own examination. You might wish to contemplate timing and adding a wellspring of fat to help ingestion.

- Use systems to make it as simple as conceivable to get more foods grown from the ground in your eating routine

- Stay away from handled food varieties and "void calories" - supplant things like chips and chocolate bars with servings of mixed greens and carrot sticks

- Keep up with this program for 30 days. You ought to find you notice you have more energy, drive, and better wellbeing.

- Utilize this new energy to work on your way of life in alternate ways!